American College
of Physicians

HOME MEDICAL GUIDE *to*

BACK PAIN

ɒ𝕜 American College of Physicians

HOME MEDICAL GUIDE *to*

BACK PAIN

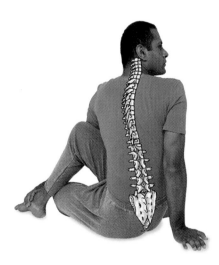

MEDICAL EDITOR
DAVID R. GOLDMANN, MD
ASSOCIATE MEDICAL EDITOR
DAVID A. HOROWITZ, MD

A DORLING KINDERSLEY BOOK

IMPORTANT

The American College of Physicians (ACP) Home Medical Guides provide general information on a wide range of health and medical topics. These books are not substitutes for medical diagnosis, and you should always consult your doctor on personal health matters before undertaking any program of therapy or treatment. Various medical organizations have different guidelines for diagnosis and treatment of the same conditions; the American College of Physicians–American Society of Internal Medicine (ACP–ASIM) has tried to present a reasonable consensus of these opinions.

Material in this book was reviewed by the ACP–ASIM for general medical accuracy and applicability in the United States; however, the information provided herein does not necessarily reflect the specific recommendations or opinions of the ACP–ASIM. The naming of any organization, product, or alternative therapy in these books is not an ACP–ASIM endorsement, and the omission of any such name does not indicate ACP–ASIM disapproval.

DORLING KINDERSLEY

LONDON, NEW YORK, AUCKLAND, DELHI,
JOHANNESBURG, MUNICH, PARIS, AND SYDNEY

DK www.dk.com

Senior Editors Jill Hamilton, Nicki Lampon
Senior Designer Jan English
DTP Design Jason Little
Editor Ashley Ren
Medical Consultant David Lennow, MD

Senior Managing Editor Martyn Page
Senior Managing Art Editor Bryn Walls

Published in the United States in 2000 by
Dorling Kindersley Publishing, Inc.
95 Madison Avenue, New York, New York 10016

2 4 6 8 10 9 7 5 3 1

Based on an original work by Professor Malcolm Jayson.

Library of Congress Catalog Card Number 99-76865
ISBN 0-7894-4166-7

Reproduced by Colourscan, Singapore
Printed and bound in the United States by Quebecor World, Taunton, Massachusetts

Contents

Introduction

Backache is not an illness in itself but a symptom. Its development means something has gone wrong somewhere, although it may not always be clear exactly what.

Most of us suffer from backache at some time or another. Usually it is an unpleasant and awkward but not desperately serious problem caused by some kind of mechanical stress or damage within the back, which gets better fairly quickly. Poor posture, excessive stresses, and wear and tear may be at least partly responsible.

It is no surprise that backache is so common. Your spine is composed of many different structures, including bones, disks, ligaments, tendons, nerves, blood vessels, and other tissues, all of which can be affected by mechanical damage resulting in backache.

In most cases, the precise cause of the problem is not important. Backache is a symptom that will clear up, and the purpose of treatment is to relieve pain and make sure that you recover as quickly as possible. Occasionally, there may be a more severe underlying cause, and detailed tests may be required to decide on the right approach to treatment. Understanding how the back works will help us protect our spines and recover more rapidly from episodes of backache.

WHO GETS BACKACHE?
Backache is a common complaint that affects almost everyone at some time in his or her life but is rarely serious.

7

This book will show you how the back works, what goes wrong, why back problems arise and how they are treated, and why and when additional tests and specialized help are necessary.

A GROWING PROBLEM

Backaches are remarkably common. At any one time, some 31,000,000 people have backaches, and about 90 percent of all people suffer at least one debilitating episode of lower back pain in their life. It affects both sexes and all ages, from children to the elderly, but it is most prevalent in middle age.

Backache is one of the most common reasons for people to take time off from work, especially in heavy manual industries. At particular risk are workers in the construction and health-care industries (for example, builders and nurses). In both cases, these workers often have to lift heavy objects in awkward positions.

It is often hard to separate cause and effect. In other words, do the stresses of the job cause the backache, or is the person unable to do heavy work because he or she already has a bad back? In many cases, back pain follows some injury or a sudden twist. Much time is now spent training workers to avoid subjecting their backs to excessive stresses.

The amount of working time lost due to back problems has increased enormously in recent years. Disability claims in the United States have increased by 14 times the rate of population growth. In fact, this dramatic rise does not mean that more people are being injured at work. There are many potential factors involved in this increase. It may relate to increased public awareness

HEAVY WORK
Lifting a heavy weight need not strain the back if the right technique is used. Always bend your hips and knees rather than your back.

Common Back Complaints

Back pain varies widely from one person to another, depending on lifestyle and occupation, but the following are common complaints:

- "I work in a factory assembling components. By the end of the day I have a terrible aching pain low down in my back, and I really don't know how much longer I can stand it."
- "It is not too bad during the day, but I wake up in the morning with a lot of pain and stiffness in my back and have to get up and move around before it eases."
- "I was just bending over to pick up a book from the floor when I felt a sudden severe pain in the bottom of my back, and I couldn't straighten up."
- "While I was working in the yard, I got a twinge of pain in my lower back. Over the next few hours the pain spread into my bottom and down the back of my leg. It really hurt, and I had to go to bed."

BACKACHE AND WORK
Standing in an awkward or static position for prolonged periods at work can exacerbate a back problem, resulting in considerable pain by the end of the day.

of health concerns as well as current systems of employee compensation. The result is a dramatic escalation in the costs of back pain to our society. The total cost now ranges from 8–20 billion dollars per year for the medical treatment provided, the benefits received, and loss of production – a phenomenal sum.

The increase in the number of people disabled by back problems has

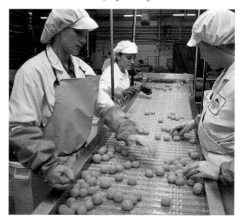

led to a complete rethinking of our approach to back pain and how it is treated. This book provides the most up-to-date views, based on the latest research on the treatment of back pain, and explains how doctors are attempting to reduce the frequency and severity of this problem.

KEY POINTS

- Backache is a symptom, not a disease.
- Acute episodes of back pain, although unpleasant, usually get better quickly.
- Backache affects more than 90 percent of the population at some time in their lives.

How the spine works

The spine, or backbone, is known medically as the vertebral column. Its role is to support the body and be capable of bending and twisting in all directions, and at the same time protect the vital structures, such as the nerves, that run through it. What's more, it has to last a lifetime.

THE FLEXIBLE BODY
The spine can bend and twist because there are flexible disks and joints that allow mobility between the vertebrae.

No engineering structure comes anywhere near meeting the exacting specifications of the spine, and it is hardly surprising that problems can arise from time to time.

THE VERTEBRAL COLUMN

The human spine consists of a column of bony blocks known as vertebrae, which sit one on top of one another to form the vertebral column. There are seven cervical vertebrae in the neck, twelve dorsal, or thoracic, vertebrae in the upper and middle back, and five lumbar vertebrae in the lower part of the spine. The fifth lumbar vertebra, known as L5, sits on the sacrum, which in turn is connected to the coccyx , or tailbone. The sacrum consists of several vertebrae that are fused together. The sacrum is joined at its edges to

The Spine – Back View

Seen from the back, the spine is a vertical column of vertebrae, attached to the pelvis at the bottom and supporting the skull at the top. The cervical vertebrae in the neck allow the skull to rotate and tilt in all directions.

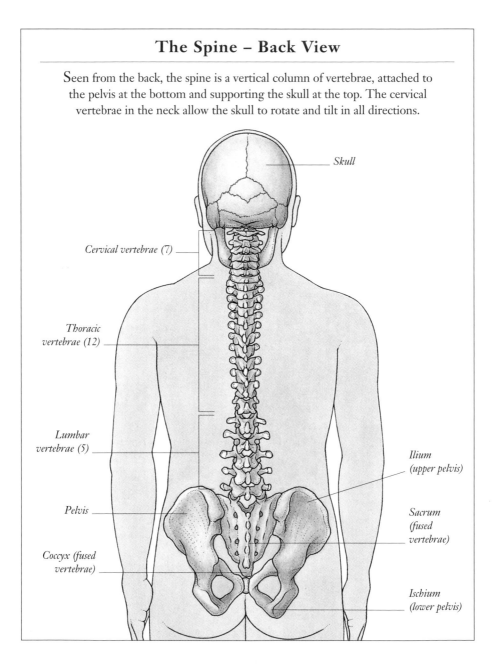

Skull

Cervical vertebrae (7)

Thoracic vertebrae (12)

Lumbar vertebrae (5)

Pelvis

Coccyx (fused vertebrae)

Ilium (upper pelvis)

Sacrum (fused vertebrae)

Ischium (lower pelvis)

The Spine – Side View

Seen from the side, the spine has a pronounced curve. The lumbar vertebrae, in the lower back, have long bony extensions to which strong muscles are attached. The sacrum and coccyx at the bottom of the spine consist of several fused vertebrae.

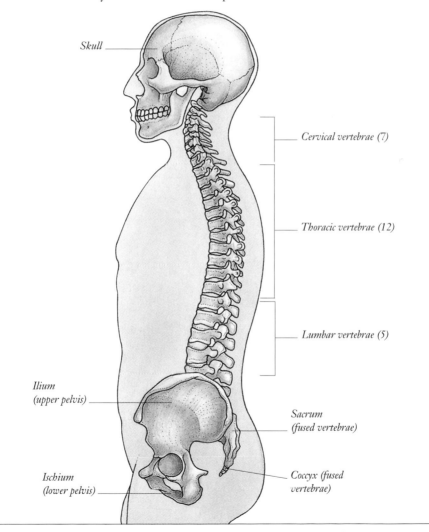

Skull

Cervical vertebrae (7)

Thoracic vertebrae (12)

Lumbar vertebrae (5)

Ilium
(upper pelvis)

Sacrum
(fused vertebrae)

Ischium
(lower pelvis)

Coccyx (fused
vertebrae)

the pelvis, the ring of bone that carries the trunk and is in turn supported by the hips.

INTERVERTEBRAL DISKS

Flexible cushions, or disks, located between the vertebrae allow the spine to bend or twist. Each disk is a flat structure with a jellylike center called the nucleus and a strong outer skin called the annulus.

The Structure of the Spine

The vertebrae are separated from one another by flexible intervertebral disks. Nerves leave the spinal cord through small bony openings between the vertebrae.

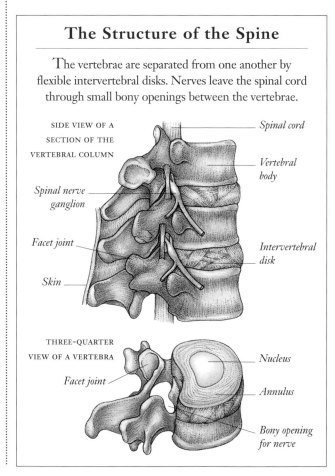

SIDE VIEW OF A SECTION OF THE VERTEBRAL COLUMN

Spinal nerve ganglion

Facet joint

Skin

Spinal cord

Vertebral body

Intervertebral disk

THREE-QUARTER VIEW OF A VERTEBRA

Facet joint

Nucleus

Annulus

Bony opening for nerve

The Nerve Network

The spinal cord is the main nerve "cable," connecting the nerves of the limbs and torso to the brain. The bony vertebral column surrounds and protects the spinal cord.

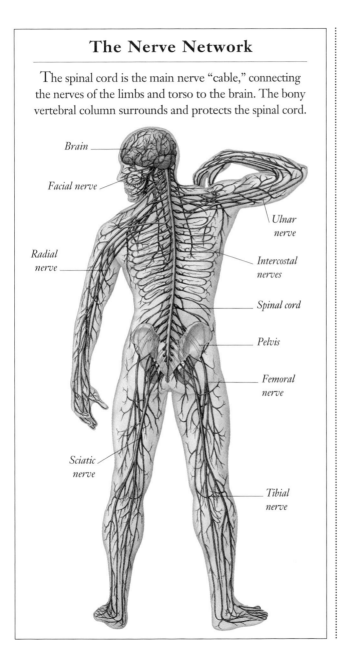

Brain

Facial nerve

Ulnar nerve

Radial nerve

Intercostal nerves

Spinal cord

Pelvis

Femoral nerve

Sciatic nerve

Tibial nerve

FACET JOINTS

The vertebrae are also joined to each other by pairs of small joints that lie at the back of the spine, one on either side. They can be affected by strain or by wear and tear. and they may develop bony swellings, causing pressure on the nerves.

NERVE NETWORK

The nervous system in some ways resembles a telephone network carrying messages from your brain to various parts of your body and back again (see p.15). Messages that pass down the nerves make muscles contract and thus control such movements as walking. Messages traveling up the nerves carry sensations, which eventually reach your brain and allow you to experience sensations such as touch and pain.

SPINAL CORD

A "cable" of nervous tissue, known as the spinal cord, extends from the brain down the spine inside the canal formed by the vertebrae. The nerve roots divide off from the spinal cord, run for short distances within the canal itself, and then exit in pairs, one on each side, from the sides of the vertebral column to supply the trunk, arms, and legs.

BACK INJURIES

If the spinal cord is damaged, its ability to transport messages between the brain and the rest of the body may be affected, leading to the loss or alteration of sensation, development of pain, and weakness of movements. This is what happens when people become paralyzed after a serious accident. The number of limbs paralyzed –

whether they can move their arms and not their legs (paraplegia), or whether all four limbs are paralyzed (quadriplegia) – depends on where the spinal cord has been damaged. If the injury is in the neck, paralysis and loss of sensation can affect both the arms and the legs.

However, if the injury is below the arm level in the thoracic or lumbar segments, then only leg muscles are affected. In most back problems, the spinal cord and nerve roots are not injured.

Pain can develop in the back itself as a result of direct injuries to the ligaments, tendons, joints, disks, and other structures in and around the vertebral column. Since the same nerves that supply these tissues also supply the legs, the pain may seem to be coming from the legs. In addition, there may be pressure directly on the nerves, also producing pain, alteration in the sense of feeling, and weakness in the legs.

It is clear that the back is a very complicated structure. When an injury has occurred, back pain may arise for several different reasons. Careful analysis is necessary in each case to determine what has happened. Fortunately, most acute episodes of back pain get better without the need for specific forms of medical intervention.

As a result, detailed tests to determine the particular injuries causing problems are generally not required. However, when symptoms are more serious and prolonged, it becomes important to determine exactly what has gone wrong. Careful examination and diagnostic tests, including some of the newer forms of imaging, may then become necessary.

KEY POINTS

- The vertebral column consists of vertebrae joined by disks and facet joints. The disk has a jellylike central nucleus and an extremely strong outer skin, the annulus.
- Back pain may arise from damage to a wide variety of structures.
- Back pain is transmitted by the nerves. The ways in which these are stimulated are complex and depend upon the particular tissue or type of nerve that has been affected.
- Since most acute episodes of back pain get better quickly, there is usually no need for detailed tests to determine the precise cause.

Common back problems

Now that we know the makeup of the spine, it is easier to understand where and why problems can arise.

NONSPECIFIC BACK PAIN

Many people who have trouble with their backs experience brief episodes of pain from which they make a full recovery. Since no firm diagnosis is made, their back pain is labeled nonspecific. Detailed tests are not necessary, and often it is not even possible to identify the particular underlying cause. Sometimes the person has tender areas over the spine or between the sacrum and the iliac bone of the pelvis. The pain may be caused by strained ligaments, tendons, disks, or other soft tissues.

Although the cause is usually uncertain, terms such as lumbosacral strain and sacroiliac strain are often used, implying that your doctor has actually made a diagnosis. The term "mechanical lower back pain" is preferable because it does not suggest that the cause of your particular problem is known. Further investigation to pinpoint the cause is necessary only if the back pain fails to improve.

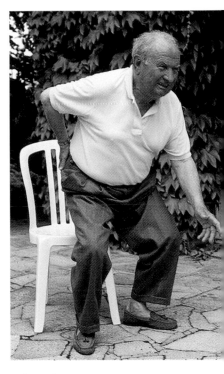

BRIEF EPISODES OF PAIN
Most back pain of sudden onset, such as that experienced when getting up from a sitting position, has no identifiable cause.

19

SLIPPED DISKS

Most people have heard of a "slipped disk," but it is an inaccurate term because disks cannot actually slip. They can wear, split, or rupture (see Protruding or herniated disk, p.47). After some particular stress on the spine, often involving bending, twisting, or lifting, the disk ruptures or prolapses, and the jellylike nucleus is squeezed out through a split in the outer annulus.

Effects of a Prolapsed Vertebral Disk

Every intervertebral disk has a fibrous outer layer, or annulus, surrounding the jellylike nucleus. Under stress, its annulus can rupture, forcing out the nucleus, which then presses on the nerve root, as this spinal cross section shows.

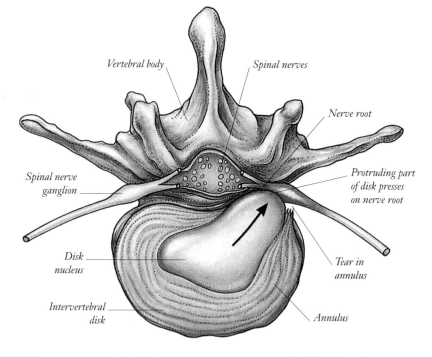

Vertebral body

Spinal nerves

Nerve root

Spinal nerve ganglion

Protruding part of disk presses on nerve root

Disk nucleus

Tear in annulus

Intervertebral disk

Annulus

We now believe that most disks that prolapse this way had previous wear and tear, and the stress on the spine triggered the problem. In other words, the disk was already abnormal and would have ruptured sooner or later. The particular stress probably just acted as the last straw.

The jellylike material, having been squeezed out, may press on the nerve running next to the disk, causing severe pain in the back that spreads down the leg and sometimes travels as far as the foot. You may feel numbness and tingling, particularly in your lower leg and foot. Some of your muscles may become weak, and the ankle-jerk reflex, tested by tapping your Achilles tendon with a reflex hammer, may be lost.

The site of these changes helps the doctor identify exactly which nerve has been irritated or injured.

The pain caused by a ruptured disk can be very severe. Usually the symptoms slowly get better and eventually disappear completely. However, once the disk has ruptured, it is permanently weak, and there is always the risk of another bout of back pain.

RADICULOPATHY (SCIATICA)

Sciatica is a nonspecific term for pain radiating down the back of the leg. It is most often caused by irritation of the lower lumbar or first sacral nerve roots. The greatest weight and bending forces are felt in the lower part of the lumbar spine. Therefore, the nerves most often damaged are the fifth lumbar nerve root, which exits between the fourth and fifth lumbar vertebrae, and the first sacral nerve root. These two join with others to form the sciatic nerve, which runs down the back of the leg to the foot. Pain arising because of damage to this nerve is commonly known as sciatica.

Sciatic Nerves

The sciatic nerves are the largest nerves in the body. They run from the lumbar and sacral regions of the spine and then down the backs of the legs.

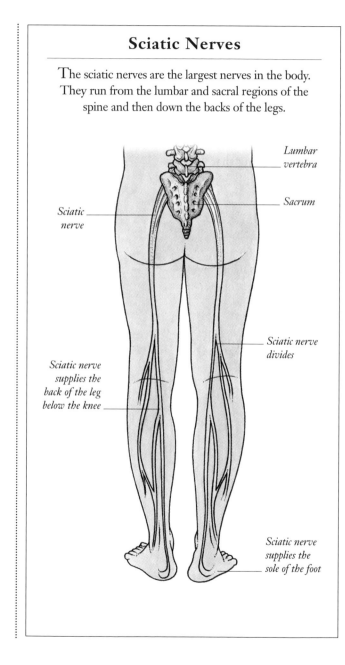

Lumbar vertebra

Sacrum

Sciatic nerve

Sciatic nerve divides

Sciatic nerve supplies the back of the leg below the knee

Sciatic nerve supplies the sole of the foot

LUMBAR SPONDYLOSIS

Spondylosis, or wear and tear of the spine, is very common. Indeed, these changes start at the age of about 25 and are present in almost all of us by the time we are middle-aged. This is one of the main reasons why athletes reach the peak of their performance in their early twenties.

The lower back bears the weight of your whole body, as well as anything that you are carrying, and does most of the bending and twisting. Consequently, wear-and-tear

---

How Wear and Tear Affects the Spine

Wear and tear in the lower part of the back, or lumbar spondylosis, is extremely common. This part of the spine bears the weight of the whole body, as well as doing most of the bending and twisting, and is therefore easily damaged.

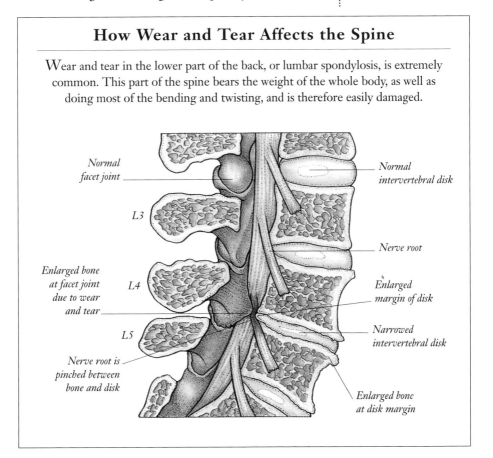

Normal facet joint

Normal intervertebral disk

L3

Nerve root

Enlarged bone at facet joint due to wear and tear

L4

Enlarged margin of disk

L5

Narrowed intervertebral disk

Nerve root is pinched between bone and disk

Enlarged bone at disk margin

changes of the spine, called lumbar spondylosis, are most common in the lumbar region.

Lumbar spondylosis is most likely to occur at the lower levels, particularly between the fourth and fifth lumbar vertebrae (L4/L5) and the fifth lumbar vertebra and the first segment of the sacrum (L5/S1), and may lead to sciatica (see p.21). It affects both the disks and the facet joints. Some material is lost from the disk and from the cartilage or gristle lining the facet joints. The bone at the margins of the disks and facet joints enlarges, making movement more limited and thus stiffening the spine. It may also press on nerves, ligaments, and other structures, causing pain.

However, this is not as depressing as it may sound. The fact that you have these wear-and-tear changes does not mean that you will necessarily suffer from backache. Many people have severe wear-and-tear changes with few or no problems, whereas others with relatively minor changes suffer incapacitating bouts of pain. It follows that wear-and-tear changes of this sort are generally of only minor significance.

LUMBAGO

One of the most common back problems is recurrent spells of acute pain, which may spread to the buttocks or to one or the other thigh. While the attack lasts, your back may also feel stiff and tender. When the symptoms are very severe the condition is called lumbago. The pain can last for a day or two or up to several weeks each time. Sometimes it just disappears completely; in other instances it may persist or recur. The symptoms are made worse by poor posture and lifting heavy weights.

PEAK PERFORMANCE
An athlete reaches his or her peak at the age of about 25, after which general wear and tear on the joints of the spine starts to affect performance.

X-rays show the presence of lumbar spondylosis, but surveys have revealed that these "wear-and-tear" changes are often found in people who do not have any symptoms. It is therefore difficult to assess the part such changes play in causing pain. As a result, the term "nonspecific back pain" is often used to describe lumbago.

NERVE PROBLEMS

Nerves get compressed or inflamed easily, both within the vertebral canal itself and as they emerge from the sides of the vertebral column, by damaged disks, facet joints, or vertebrae. When a nerve is compressed, its ability to pass messages is affected. When this happens, you may experience pain or a sensation of numbness or tingling in the area supplied by the nerve, and the muscles that it controls in your leg or foot may become weak. The spinal cord transmits these sensations to the brain, and the effect is like interference on a telephone wire, producing poor-quality sound. Research indicates, however, that it is much more complicated than that.

Changes within the spinal cord itself can affect the pain message. This may explain why some patients continue to experience widespread pain and symptoms long after the original nerve damage has healed and there is little evidence of any problem.

COCCYDYNIA

Coccydynia is pain at the tail end of the spine, or the coccyx. Usually, unless the pain is due to injury, no cause is found. A soft cushion ring or a gel cushion may be used to make sitting more comfortable, but the pain usually goes away by itself in time.

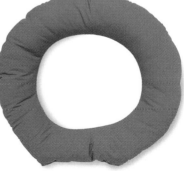

RELIEVING THE PRESSURE
A soft ring-shaped cushion will make sitting more comfortable if you are suffering from an injury to the coccyx.

NECK PROBLEMS

This section will deal only briefly with common neck disorders. The neck shares the same basic structure as the rest of the spine and is therefore also prone to disk problems and wear-and-tear changes.

While pain in the lower back commonly shoots down the legs, neck pain may involve the shoulders and arms. For uncomplicated neck problems, treatment with rest, pain medication, and perhaps physical therapy usually suffices. A padded neck collar may be helpful to make sure that the neck is properly supported and rested.

ACUTE STIFF NECK SYNDROME

Many people have had the experience of waking up with a stiff and painful neck, and often there seems to be no particular reason. Movement may be possible only in one direction, and the muscles of the lower neck may be tender. There are no other problems with the rest of the back or with the arms or legs. The pain is associated with muscle spasm and will abate with a collar and pain medication in three to four days.

WHIPLASH

This is common after a car accident, when the sudden impact gives no time for muscles to brace, and the head moves like a pendulum on the neck. In the simplest cases only ligaments in the neck are sprained, and the pain and stiffness that result are caused by the neck muscles going into spasm as a protective mechanism. If there are no other problems, a soft collar, pain medication, and, in some cases, physical therapy are all that are needed. For most patients, early return to normal activity gives the best results. In some cases, pain persists for longer

How Whiplash Occurs

Whiplash injury commonly results from a front- or rear-impact car accident. The neck is forced suddenly forward and then backward, spraining the ligaments.

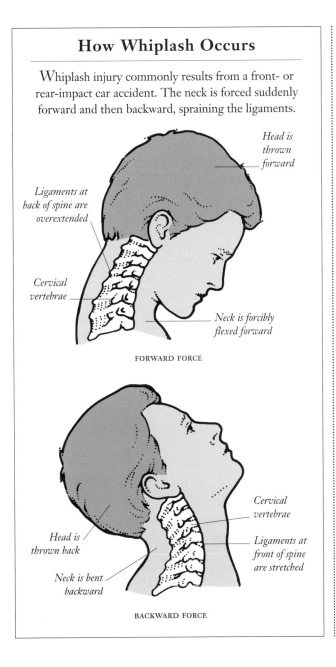

Head is thrown forward

Ligaments at back of spine are overextended

Cervical vertebrae

Neck is forcibly flexed forward

FORWARD FORCE

Cervical vertebrae

Ligaments at front of spine are stretched

Head is thrown back

Neck is bent backward

BACKWARD FORCE

than six weeks, and it may be that the initial injury was more serious, causing damage to the disks or other structures, and has led to nerves being damaged or trapped. Facet joints are a common source of pain from whiplash injuries. More detailed investigation is needed. When pain remains severe for several months, it becomes more likely that there will be continuing disability.

DISK PROBLEMS IN THE NECK

Disks can also prolapse in the neck, although this is less common than in the lower back. The neck is extremely stiff, and pain may shoot down one arm. Strength, sensation, and reflexes in the arm may be lost. In the majority of cases, the pain will ease with rest, pain relief medication, and traction if necessary. Physical therapy to strengthen the neck muscles is also useful. Facet joint or epidural injections may also be helpful.

USING A NECK COLLAR
After a whiplash injury, a neck collar provides support and restricts excessive movement until muscle spasm has eased.

CERVICAL SPONDYLOSIS

Wear-and-tear problems in the neck are known as cervical spondylosis. They may cause no problems at all or lead to neck pain with headache and/or arm pain. Neck movements are reduced, and some patients have a tender spot in the trapezius muscle, which lies between the neck and the shoulders. As with disk problems in the neck, the arms may become weak and lose their reflexes. There may be tingling or pins and needles in the arms. In the most serious cases, the distorted bone and ligaments can press on the spinal cord, affecting control of the arms and legs, or on an artery in the region called the vertebral artery, leading to dizziness, buzzing in the ear, and pain behind the eyes. Many people who have cervical spondylosis also have lower back pain. The principles of treatment are the same: use of a soft collar for a short time, physical therapy, anti-inflammatory drugs, pain relief medication, and early mobilization. Surgery may be necessary for a small proportion of patients.

KEY POINTS

- Disks do not slip, but they can rupture.
- Sciatica is caused by damage to the nerves that join to form the sciatic nerve running down the lower limb.
- Wear and tear, or spondylosis, of the spine is very common as you get older, but it does not inevitably lead to back pain.
- Neck problems have many similarities to back pain.

Treating back pain: the first steps

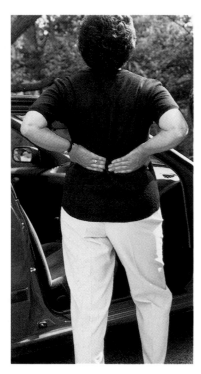

SIMPLE BACK PAIN
Some back pain, such as the discomfort experienced after a long drive, may disappear a few minutes after stretching your back and moving around.

Most of us get sudden episodes of pain in the back from time to time, usually lasting only a day or so. Apart from being careful, you do not need to do anything about it, and it is soon forgotten. Some people, however, may develop more severe attacks of pain that limit their activity and ability to work.

Despite all our modern technology, in many cases we cannot determine the exact source of back pain. It could well be the result of some damage to the ligaments, muscles, or other soft tissues, but often your doctor may be unable to diagnose the precise cause. The good news, however, is that usually it does not matter, since most of these acute attacks of back pain will get better without treatment.

The most common problem is simple backache, in which the pain is confined to the back or may spread down into the buttock or upper thigh. Sometimes it may extend down the leg, resulting in sciatica, commonly caused by radiculopathy. Pressure on one of the nerve roots may come from a damaged disk or other structures, causing pain and sometimes numbness and tingling running down your leg. Symptoms of radiculopathy suggest that there has been some nerve damage and that recovery is likely to be slow.

Occasionally, a person may develop more severe symptoms of a back problem and should be seen promptly by a specialist. This will be necessary for any person who experiences problems controlling the bladder or bowel, numbness in the groin or rectal area, or severe leg weakness, all of which could indicate more severe nerve damage.

ASSESSING THE PROBLEM

Usually, when you have an acute back problem, the physician treating you will ask for details about how and when the pain started and what has happened since and will perform a physical examination. Questions that you may be asked include:

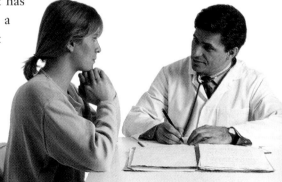

- Is the pain confined to one area only or is it more generalized?
- Does the pain shoot or spread to another part of the body, for example, to the leg?
- Did the pain begin suddenly or gradually? If gradually, over what period of time?
- Was the onset associated with any activity?
- Does anything make the pain worse?
- What is the pain like first thing in the morning?
- Are you otherwise well? Have you lost weight or do you have a cough or other problems?

VISITING A SPECIALIST
If your back pain is severe, you will be referred to a specialist for assessment.

31

Back pain that started while lifting a heavy object, that is sharp and limited to a small area, and that gets better with rest is likely to be uncomplicated, and the pain should go away quickly. However, if the pain developed gradually over many months, does not seem to be linked with movement, and becomes more severe, and if there are other problems, such as weight loss, the cause may be more serious, and special diagnostic tests may be necessary.

You may be sent for an X-ray, but usually this is not necessary. Although the X-ray may show that you have some wear-and-tear changes, these features are common

Back Examination

If your back pain does not clear up of its own accord, you may be sent to a specialist for further examination. The specialist, or your primary physician, may carry out some or all of the following:

- Look for signs of curvature and observe the way that your back bends and how you walk.
- Feel your back for tender spots or areas.
- Perform the straight-leg raising test. The doctor lifts each leg straight up while you are lying flat on your back. If there is a problem with the lower nerve roots, this will cause pain.
- Perform the femoral stretch test. The doctor places you lying down on your front, then slowly bends each knee in turn. If there is a problem with the femoral nerve, or upper lumbar nerve roots, this will cause pain.
- Look for loss of sensation or weakness in the legs.
- Check your reflexes.

in people without backache and do not have much influence on treatment. Each X-ray exposes you to radiation, and, consequently, X-rays are usually reserved for people with severe back pain that has not responded to simple treatment and for those who have more complicated back problems or history of trauma.

You are unlikely to need more detailed types of imaging, such as magnetic resonance imaging (MRI) or computerized tomography (CT) scans (see pp.56–57).

HOW IS IT TREATED?

For most people with acute back pain, only very simple treatment is needed:

• Take simple pain relievers such as acetaminophen or ibuprofen. When used appropriately, these pills have few side effects and are usually all you need. You can ask your doctor for stronger pain medication, available by prescription, if you feel that you need it.

• A short period of bed rest is helpful, but too much rest can actually aggravate the problem. If you are in severe pain, you should rest lying flat with a pillow placed under your knees for a couple of days. After that, you should start to move around again, taking care to protect your back but with an eye toward returning to normal physical activity.

• A cold pack, such as a bag of ice, against your back may help relieve the pain. Alternatively, you can try heat in the form of a heating pad or a hot shower. However, neither is likely to make any long-term difference.

For most people, simple remedies such as these are enough, and the pain will usually clear up within a few days or a couple of weeks. You should try to get back to normal physical activity as soon as possible.

It is important that you pay attention to the advice in the chapter on how to protect your back; this will reduce your chances of having another attack in the future (see Protecting your back, pp.37–44).

You may, however, find that your pain does not disappear completely. If you still have a problem after about four to six weeks, you may be referred to a specialist. This might be:

BACK THERAPY
Trained therapists can assess back conditions and ease pain by massage and exercise.

- A doctor with special expertise in the appropriate treatment techniques;
- A physical therapist;
- An osteopath;
- A chiropractor.

Physical therapy is the most traditional form of therapy, and it usually involves the combination of heat, gentle massage, and exercise to help someone regain his or her normal movement, strength, and flexibility. Many physical therapists may also be trained in the methods of joint manipulation.

Both osteopathic and chiropractic treatments tend to concentrate on joint manipulation. All therapists will give advice on the care and protection of the back. In practice, however, it is doubtful whether there is much difference between these techniques because, in all three cases, the principles lying behind treatment are the same and include mobilization with exercises of various types and manipulation.

The treatment for sciatica, which is commonly caused by radiculopathy (see p.21), also involves pain medication such as analgesics, rest, and mobilization, but progress is often much slower. Sometimes people with this particular problem must have surgery in order to relieve the pressure on the nerve. More information on persistent back pain is given in the next two chapters.

MANIPULATION THERAPY
Manipulating the joints of the spine can help restore mobility.

RECURRENT BACK PAIN

The natural history of most acute back episodes is recovery, usually within a few days but sometimes taking a week or even two.

People with a history of back pain are likely to develop further episodes in the future. Sometimes recurrences are the result of an accident or lifting an exceptionally heavy load, but for many people acute relapses may be precipitated by trivial physical activities. Understanding how the back works and minimizing stresses on the spine, together with improvement in physical fitness, will help prevent further relapses.

KEY POINTS

- Most acute back pain is simple backache. A small proportion of people develop sciatica, and a few have more complicated problems.
- Simple backache usually responds to pain relief medication, a short period of bed rest if necessary, and then early physical activity and return to work.
- If there is no improvement, you may be referred to a therapist or a specialist, who may undertake further tests and treatment.

Protecting your back

Some people who have an underlying back weakness go through repeated bouts of back pain, often because of a combination of poor posture and excessive stresses on the back.

We now know how different positions and loads affect the back and may lead to back problems, but you can teach yourself how to minimize the stresses you place on your back. These lessons are actually valuable for all of us, but they are especially important for anyone who is susceptible to back pain.

IMPROVING YOUR POSTURE

How we stand and sit is important and may greatly affect our ability to cope with back pain. Being careful about your posture will minimize a lot of stresses on your spine. Poor posture can stretch the spinal ligaments and, as a result, cause aching and stiffness in your back. Either forward-flexed posture or leaning forward when you are seated places high force on the lumbar disks and may cause injury. The following tips will help you improve your posture:

• Stand upright with your back straight and your head facing forward; avoid slouching.

• When you are working at a bench, make sure that it is high enough for you to stand in a comfortable

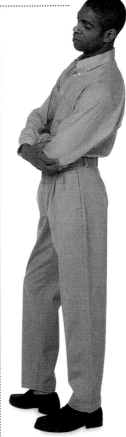

POOR POSTURE
Standing poorly, with a curved spine, will eventually lead to back pain. Always stand upright with your weight balanced evenly on both feet.

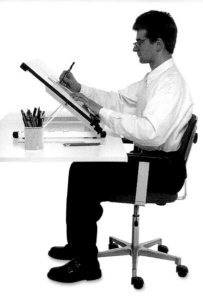

working posture and, in particular, that you can stand upright.

- A desk should be of sufficient height and have enough leg space so that you are close enough to sit upright and work comfortably. You should have plenty of room under the work surface so that you can get close to your work without having to bend forward and your legs and feet are free to move.
- Keeping still in one position for a long time is an important cause of aching and stiffness.
- When sitting at a desk, make sure that you can sit upright with a support in the small of your back.

THE WORK STATION
Be sure that you can get close to your work without having to bend forward. It is also important to sit upright when working at a desk. If necessary, use a raised surface, as this man is doing.

EXAMINING YOUR SHOES

Women who experience back pain should not wear high heels. They tip the lower part of your body forward and you then arch your upper body backward to compensate, putting stress on your back. It is better to wear shoes that do not have hard leather soles. Hard soles send shock waves up through your skeleton as your heels strike the ground and thereby aggravate back problems. Cushioned soles and heels or shock-absorbing insoles can reduce this effect and often make walking much easier. Sneakers or other soft-soled supportive shoes are particularly recommended because they are comfortable and minimize these sudden shock waves.

DRIVING COMFORTABLY

Backache is common to all of us who spend long periods driving. Anyone who is prone to backache can experience particular problems. In recent years, car manufacturers have paid much more attention to the design of the car seat and the driver's position in order to minimize backache. However, we still often find seats that are poorly designed, holding the back in a rounded position. Sitting for a long time in this posture can cause excruciating back pain. The best car seats have a built-in adjustable lumbar support, and the height, seat, and back angles can be altered to suit the individual driver. The foot controls should be squarely in front of your feet and not at an angle, which causes constant spine-twisting. Adequate side mirrors will help you avoid having to twist around, and power steering lessens the strain on your spine when you are maneuvering the car at low speeds.

SITTING INCORRECTLY
Avoid sitting on a stool with your back bent forward. It will aggravate backache and cause stiffness.

SITTING PROPERLY

Many chairs are poorly designed. Often the worst are low armchairs and easy chairs that look temptingly soft but hold your back in a rounded position, causing severe aching and stiffness. Perching on a stool with your back bent forward often aggravates backache and stiffness, and you should avoid it if you can. You will be most comfortable in an upright chair that supports your lower back, maintaining the normal slightly inward curve of the lumbar part of your spine.

Alternatively, place a back rest or lumbar roll behind the small of your back to obtain adequate support. If necessary, you can make your own lumbar support using a small cushion or a rolled-up towel.

SITTING CORRECTLY
Try to sit upright with the natural curve of your back maintained and both feet flat on the floor.

39

MONITORING MOVEMENTS

Bending forward and twisting combined with carrying a heavy load are the most likely movements to stress your spine and cause back problems. Avoiding this kind of stress is important for all of us, but especially for anyone with a back problem.

SAFE CARRYING
Never carry anything that is too heavy for you. Always keep the objects close to your body and try to keep loads evenly balanced.

LIFTING CORRECTLY

Many back problems develop during lifting. Frequently this happens when load-bearing is combined with bending forward and twisting the spine. There are some simple practical guidelines that help protect the back and reduce the risk of back trouble.

IS THE OBJECT TOO HEAVY?

The first priority when lifting is to decide whether the load is too heavy or bulky to move on your own. There are no hard and fast rules about the maximum weight that can be lifted safely. Much depends on the circumstances; the position that is required; the size, shape, and weight of the object; and on your own strength and health.

The strain on your spine is much greater if the object is held at arm's length rather than close to your body. Someone with back problems can carry much less than someone without these problems.

Grip the object firmly with your palms and the base of your fingers and thumbs rather than with your fingers alone. Heavy objects should not be lifted above shoulder level because it places tremendous strain on the spine.

How to Lift Objects: The Kinetic Method

Lifting incorrectly is the root of many back problems. Follow the instructions below to minimize the risk of straining the ligaments in the back, which causes acute back pain.

STEP 1

The right way to lift is to place your feet apart, at right angles to each other, and with the front foot pointing in the direction in which the object is to be moved. This puts you in a stable position and prevents you from twisting your back in the process of lifting and then pushing off.

STEP 2

Crouch down, bending your hips and knees but keeping your back straight. Your whole spine may be inclined forward, but it is important to avoid bending your back. In this position your knees are well apart, and the object is positioned between them and kept close to your body. You can get a good, firm grip, and the lift is performed using your leg muscles. Make sure not to hold your breath while lifting.

STEP 3

Once you are upright, you should carry the load close to your body without twisting your back. Put it down carefully, using the same procedure in reverse.

This is known as the kinetic method of lifting. Many industries train their workers to use this technique automatically, but it should be the lifting method used by everybody.

41

SLEEPING PROPERLY

Many people get backaches from their beds. Such backaches are often the result of a poor-quality mattress and box spring, which sag under the weight of the body. Furthermore, most of us sleep on our sides, and a sagging bed therefore produces a sideways bend in the back that may lead to considerable aching and stiffness. You can usually prevent this by sleeping on a bed that does not sag as easily. The ideal bed is one with a firm, well-sprung mattress and box spring. The mattress does not need to be hard.

In fact, it may be a mistake to buy a very firm, hard bed in the belief that it is good for your back because it might be so uncomfortable that you do not sleep well. When you are choosing a bed, spend some time lying on it to be sure that it is firm but comfortable.

Unfortunately, a well-sprung, quality bed can be very expensive. An alternative, which is almost as effective, is to place a firm board on top of the box spring and underneath the mattress. It should run the full length of the bed and be thick enough not to bend under the weight of your body. A sheet of plywood about three-quarters of an inch (2 cm) thick is a good choice for this purpose.

USING JUST ONE PILLOW

You should lie with your body as straight as possible so that neither your spine nor your neck bends to the side during the night. Using too many pillows causes your neck to twist sideways, and this misalignment may lead to acute pain. It is usually better to use only one pillow so that your head and neck are in line with the rest of your body when you lie on your side.

STAYING IN SHAPE

If you are overweight, you are putting additional strain on your back, and you may also have poor posture. Losing weight is important not only for your back but also because it is good for your general health. Physical fitness and exercise form an important part of prevention and treatment if you are prone to back problems. Doctors strongly believe that exercise helps prevent back pain by increasing the ability of the trunk to handle lifting or carrying loads.

There are many suitable types of exercise for people with back problems, such as aerobics, weight-training, and simple stretching and bending exercises (see pp.60–62). Staying in shape and strengthening the muscles in your spine are both very important.

Unfortunately, some exercises can make back pain worse. If you have a back problem, it is important to be careful and concentrate on doing the kinds of exercise that are designed for strengthening the back and stomach muscles, rather than those aimed at forcing back movements.

STAYING IN SHAPE
Your back will benefit from regular exercise and stretching, which help keep the spine muscles strong and flexible, thereby preventing damage.

43

KEY POINTS

- Good posture is important for preventing backache. Change positions and shift weight frequently.
- The shoes we wear and the chairs we sit in can also affect our backs. Avoid high heels and sagging chairs.
- When lifting an object, follow the kinetic method of lifting and avoid lifting very heavy objects.
- Make sure that your bed has a firm but comfortable mattress, and avoid using too many pillows.

What causes persistent back pain?

Some people suffer from persistent or chronic back pain and need careful evaluation to find out why. Once the cause is identified, an appropriate treatment program can be planned.

By far the most common cause of chronic back pain is some mechanical disorder in the back. However, in a small proportion of people, pain is the result of inflammatory diseases, bone disorders, tumors, or problems in the abdomen or pelvis.

MECHANICAL BACK PAIN

Many people suffer persistent pain in the back, which may spread into the buttock or leg. Often, the pain is aggravated by physical activity and by certain postures. The spine is a very complicated structure, and many different things can go wrong. The following are common causes of chronic mechanical back pain.

AGGRAVATING FACTORS
A day's digging can exacerbate back pain from strained muscles and ligaments.

LUMBAR SPONDYLOSIS

X-rays of the back frequently show signs of aging changes in the intervertebral disks and facet joints. Indeed, they are present in almost every older person. Although people with these aging changes get backache more often than those without, there is no clear-cut correlation between wear and tear and the symptoms of back pain. Although X-rays may show evidence of severe wear and tear, the person may be symptom-free. For this reason, signs of wear and tear in the spine should be treated with caution. Just because you have them and also have backache does not mean that the changes are necessarily the cause of the symptoms. Nor does it mean that someone who has these changes but is not experiencing a backache is bound to develop back problems or become disabled in the future.

In lumbar spondylosis, pain is felt across the lower back and is sometimes worse on one side than on the other.

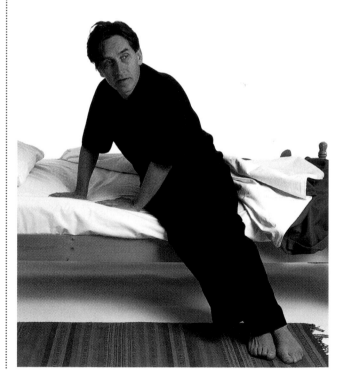

EARLY MORNING STIFFNESS
People who have lumbar spondylosis often stiffen up after spending a long time in one position. This is especially common when getting up out of bed in the mornings.

The pain increases with physical exercise and bending and is relieved by rest. However, some people tend to stiffen when they stay in one position for an extended length of time. This may be most noticeable first thing in the morning or after prolonged sitting in an easy chair. The pain can spread to one or the other buttock and sometimes to the back of the thigh.

Back movements are usually limited, but often this affects only certain types of movements, while other movements are relatively free.

PROTRUDING OR HERNIATED DISK

Under stress, a disk can rupture, usually backward and to one side, causing it to press on a nerve. This leads to pain in the back, and if the pain spreads farther down into the leg, it is called sciatica. When the disk prolapses, the person may develop radiculopathy (see p.21). In most cases, the disk was already showing marked evidence of wear and tear damage and was seriously weakened. Some particular stress precipitated the development of the rupture that was about to occur. The problem may lead to chronic pain and disability.

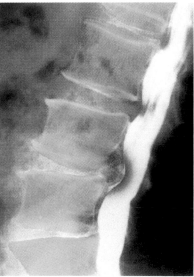

A person who is suffering from a herniated disk may experience pain in the buttock that spreads down the back or outside of the thigh to the back of the calf and sometimes into the foot, usually on the top or outer side. Pain is frequently accompanied by a sensation of tingling, or pins and needles, known technically as "paresthesia." There may also be a feeling of numbness.

PAINFUL PRESSURE
In this color-enhanced X-ray image, an intervertebral disk has herniated, pressing on the spinal cord (shown as white) at the point highlighted in pink.

47

The doctor's examination may reveal evidence that the nerve is trapped or irritated. When the leg is kept straight and lifted upward, there is a lot of pain, and movement is limited. There may be weakness of certain movements of the foot, and the ankle reflex can be lost. The feeling in the area of the damaged nerve may also be reduced.

HYPERMOBILITY

Some people have remarkably flexible joints. They can bend forward with the legs straight to place the palms of their hands flat on the ground. The joints of the arms and legs can bend to a remarkable degree. This flexibility is known as hypermobility. Many athletes, gymnasts, and professional dancers are hyper-mobile; it is this facility that enables them to undertake physical activities far beyond most of us.

In later years, hypermobility predisposes the individual to the development of joint symptoms. Ironically, in some people, back motion may remain normal in spite of pain. With the passage of time, hypermobility can become a significant cause of back problems.

INHERITED VARIATIONS IN THE SPINE

We are all different shapes and sizes, and our spines vary accordingly. Some people are born with an extra lumbar vertebra or one too few, or one or more vertebrae may be abnormally shaped. These variations are usually unimportant and do not cause pain.

SPONDYLOLISTHESIS AND SPONDYLOLYSIS

Sometimes one vertebra slips forward or back on top of the one below because of a weakness in the supporting

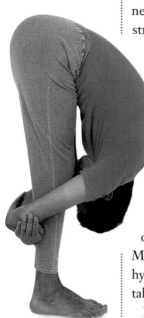

FLEXIBLE JOINTS
Hypermobility may predispose a person to joint problems in later life due to excessive wear and tear and over-stretched ligaments.

arches of the vertebral column. This condition is known as spondylolisthesis and can cause pain because it results in overstretching of nerves or ligaments.

The slippage may be the result of failure of the supporting bones in the spine to develop properly, wear and tear of the vertebrae themselves, or a fracture. When a stress fracture develops in a particular portion of the vertebra but no displacement occurs, the condition is called spondylolysis.

SPINAL STENOSIS

The nerve roots run down from the spinal cord within the vertebral column and then emerge from the sides of the vertebral column through narrow openings. Each opening is known as a foramen; two or more, as foramina. The nerve roots then run down into the legs.

We all have spinal canals and foramina of different sizes and shapes. Some are smaller than others, putting the nerves that run through them at particular risk of getting compressed.

Narrowing of the central canal of the vertebral column is known as central stenosis. This condition may lead to pain, numbness, and tingling in the legs, any of which symptoms may develop when walking and are relieved by rest or bending forward. The pain is intensified by arching backward. These symptoms are similar to the leg problems that are associated with poor blood supply to the legs.

When narrowing affects the foramina through which the nerve roots emerge, patients may develop persistent, unremitting sciatica-type pain. This is known as foraminal stenosis. Surgery to relieve this type of nerve pressure can be very effective.

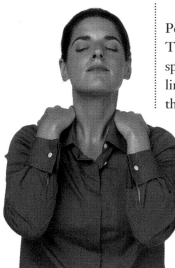

A Painful Neck
Back pain that spreads into the neck area is one of the most common symptoms of fibromyalgia.

FIBROMYALGIA

People with fibromyalgia develop a range of symptoms. They experience widespread pain across the back spreading up the back of the chest into the neck and the limbs. They often have tender points, especially over the sacroiliac joints, the shoulder blades, the inside and outside of the elbows and knees, and elsewhere. Frequently, a variety of detailed tests have failed to pinpoint a particular abnormality.

Many people with fibromyalgia are frequently anxious and depressed, and they often feel tired and listless. It is often difficult for doctors to decide whether the persistent pain has led to the patient's depression or whether the depression has caused them to feel the pain more severely. The explanation may lie in changes in the way pain sensations are transmitted in the spinal cord.

Many people who suffer from fibromyalgia sleep poorly and wake up feeling unrefreshed with generalized aches, pains, and stiffness. Some research suggests that poor sleep rhythm may actually be responsible for the condition. People with fibromyalgia may often have other problems as well, such as irritable bowel syndrome and migraine.

OTHER CAUSES OF BACK PAIN

Although most backaches are the result of mechanical disorders such as those that have already been described, in a small proportion of people it is a symptom of some other illness. For this reason, you should always be thoroughly checked by a doctor, particularly when back pain develops for the first time or when its nature suddenly changes.

INFECTION

Occasionally people with severe back problems are found to have chronic infection in the disks or elsewhere, but this is very uncommon.

ANKYLOSING SPONDYLITIS

This is an inflammatory form of arthritis in which the effects are concentrated in the back. Sometimes it can attack the joints of the arms and legs and occasionally other body tissues. Most often it starts in young male adults, but it may occur in women and can start at any age. The initial problems appear in the joints between the sacrum and the pelvis (sacroiliac joints) and may then spread up the spine. As it advances, it can cause stiffening of the back and a pronounced stoop, and in severe cases the spine may end up completely rigid.

Unlike people who have mechanical backache, those with ankylosing spondylitis may find that their pain and stiffness are aggravated by rest and relieved by exercise. They often toss and turn in bed and wake up in the morning aching and stiff. Many get up during the night and do some physical exercise to obtain relief. As the condition worsens, the aching and stiffness may last longer through the day. Your doctor will examine you and probably order blood tests and X-rays to confirm thediagnosis.

BONE DISORDERS

The skeleton provides the scaffolding that supports the soft tissues of the body. Unlike a metal framework, bone is a living material in which the constituents are constantly being renewed. There are several types of disease that lead to weakening and deformity of the bone and may make you more prone to fractures:

The Effects of Osteoporosis

Thinning of the interior of the bones makes them lighter, more fragile, brittle, and more prone to fracture. When the bones of the spine are affected, the weakened vertebrae may become crushed, causing pain and loss of height.

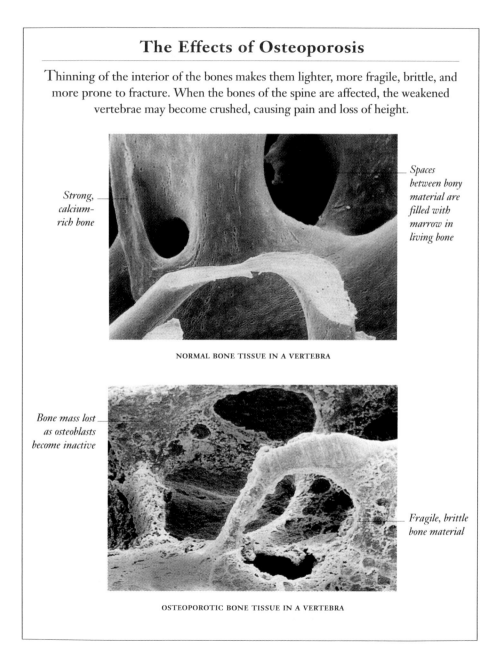

Strong, calcium-rich bone

Spaces between bony material are filled with marrow in living bone

NORMAL BONE TISSUE IN A VERTEBRA

Bone mass lost as osteoblasts become inactive

Fragile, brittle bone material

OSTEOPOROTIC BONE TISSUE IN A VERTEBRA

- **Osteoporosis** This is a common form of bone disease. It most commonly affects women after menopause, when hormonal changes lead to weakening of their bone structure, but it can affect men as well. Some people develop osteoporosis as a result of hormonal disorders such as Cushing's disease or as a complication of treatment with certain steroid drugs.

  When the bone is weakened, tiny fractures occur very easily and the vertebrae become compressed. Some people experience repeated attacks of severe back pain as a result and gradually develop a stoop.

  The loss of height and severe forward bending that often affects older women after menopause is usually caused by osteoporosis.

- **Osteomalacia** People who have been diagnosed with osteomalacia lack calcium and vitamin D. The lack can be the result of a diet low in dairy products, failure to absorb calcium from the bowel, or lack of sunlight. Their bones become progressively weaker so that they are more prone to fractures and pain.

- **Paget's disease of the bone** This condition, which most commonly affects the elderly, causes normal bone to break down and be replaced by abnormal bone that grows very quickly. The new bone is weaker, thicker, and distorted. It may fracture easily or press on nerves and ligaments, causing tenderness and pain.

TUMORS

Sometimes back pain can be caused by a tumor developing in the back or spreading from elsewhere. Although it is a rare cause of backache, the possibility has to be ruled out, and it is therefore important to have a thorough medical assessment.

REFERRED PAIN

This is the term doctors use to describe pain that you feel in your back but which actually has its origin somewhere else in your body.

Not all back pain is caused by problems in and around the spine. Stomach ulcers, gynecological problems, and some other conditions can result in pressure on nerves and cause back pain. When there is some link between bouts of pain and a woman's menstrual cycle, doctors will consider whether there may be a gynecological cause. Sometimes it is not obvious that the problem is actually coming from the abdomen or pelvis.

KEY POINTS

- There are a number of medical conditions that cause back pain, including many mechanical disorders.
- Back pain can also be a symptom of a condition such as inflammation, infection, bone disorders, and referred pain.
- Changes associated with the aging process can cause back problems in the elderly.
- In women after menopause, osteoporosis can cause back pain and bending of the spine.

Treating persistent back pain

Treatment for persistent back pain may include a special exercise program, drug therapy, or surgery. It is important to get your doctor's assessment of the problem before deciding on the appropriate treatment.

CLINICAL EXAMINATION
Your doctor will carry out a thorough physical examination, which may include a straight-leg raising test, in order to make a diagnosis of back pain.

MAKING A DIAGNOSIS

A diagnosis can generally be made by clinical examination alone, but additional tests may be necessary in some cases.

YOUR MEDICAL HISTORY

For your doctor, the most important part of assessing your back problem is finding out from you exactly how the pain started and what has happened since, together with other medical details. You will then have a physical examination. That may be all that is necessary.

BLOOD TESTS

Most backaches have a mechanical cause, and the results of blood tests are normal. However, such tests can be useful if inflammatory and other possible causes of back pain are being investigated. In particular, ankylosing spondylitis (see p.51) is associated with a certain white blood cell type, HLA-B27. If this is not present when your blood test results come back, you are less likely to have this condition. A result that shows the presence of HLA-B27, however, does not prove that you actually have ankylosing spondylitis, since this white cell type is found in about 8 percent of healthy people who do not have this condition.

X-RAYS

Vast numbers of spinal X-rays are taken, but the majority are unnecessary. The only people who need them are those with severe back pain that has not improved with simple treatment and those with complicated problems or trauma. Unnecessary X-rays are avoided because each involves some, albeit slight, exposure to radiation.

CT SCANNING

CT means computerized tomography. CT scans enable doctors to use X-rays to obtain a clearer view of the internal structures of the vertebral column. In particular, the inner outlines of the bony structures can be examined, and some details of the disks can be seen.

ONLY WHEN NECESSARY
Many X-rays are taken of the spine, but these usually give little information about the cause of a problem.

MAGNETIC RESONANCE IMAGING

MRI involves the use of very strong magnetic fields rather than X-rays. It is particularly good for studying the nerves, ligaments, and disks within the bony structures.

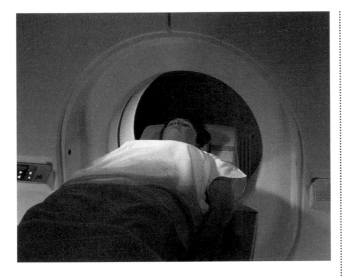

CT SCANNING
A patient enters a computerized tomography scanner, which will give a detailed picture of the structures in the spine and may help explain this person's symptoms.

LIMITATIONS OF CT AND MRI

These imaging methods are widely available. However, it is not always clear who can actually benefit from being scanned using this technology. As with X-rays of the back, the changes that they reveal often correlate poorly with symptoms.

MYELOGRAMS

When we look at X-rays of the spine, we are actually studying shadows of the bones. We cannot see the soft tissues, such as the nerves and disks within the spine.

In a myelogram, dye that is opaque to X-rays is injected into the spinal column. When a disk has ruptured, the column of dye will be indented where the disk presses into the spinal column. The exact location of the damaged disk can then be identified on the X-ray. Myelograms are rarely performed today because CT scanning or MRI are generally used instead.

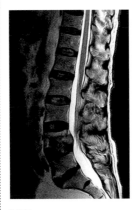

MRI
As this MRI scan of the spine shows, the technique produces a high-quality image of the vertebrae, disks, and muscles.

NONDRUG TREATMENTS

The treatment of chronic back pain depends on whether it results from mechanical problems, the most common cause, or from some other disorder.

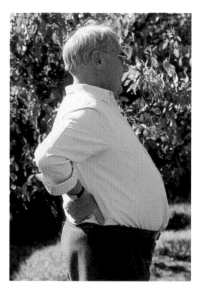

LONG-TERM DISCOMFORT
Back problems frequently affect people who are overweight. Losing weight and taking up a carefully tailored exercise program will help restore normal mobility.

CARING FOR YOUR BACK

Physical activity is good for people with chronic back problems. You should try to keep active and to exercise, although you do need to take some sensible precautions. You have to be careful, for example, to avoid overstressing your back and to be aware of your posture when standing, sitting, and lifting. A job lifting heavy loads is not appropriate for you.

PHYSICAL THERAPY

Views on treatment have changed dramatically in the last few years. We now believe that the principal role of the physical therapist is to get you mobile again and restore you to normal levels of activity as soon as possible. It is important that you be referred to a physical therapist if your back problem has lasted more than a few weeks and is in danger of becoming chronic.

The physical therapist will teach you how your back works, what can go wrong, and how to protect the back against excessive stress, and will demonstrate exercises aimed at restoring your mobility so that you can start to function normally again.

The exercise program will normally be tailored to fit your individual needs and will include exercises to strengthen your back and abdominal muscles, together with leg stretches and aerobic conditioning.

Sometimes the physical therapist will apply various forms of heat, such as an infrared lamp or short-wave diathermy. Other aids include ice packs or cooling aerosol sprays, ultrasound, and massage. Such treatments do not cure the long-term problem, but they can be extremely soothing and relaxing. Their special value is often seen as preliminary to other forms of treatment such as exercises, which otherwise would be very painful.

Traction, like many other back pain treatments, has been used since ancient times. The idea is to stretch damaged joints and relieve pressure on damaged nerves. It helps at the time, but its long-term value is doubtful, and its use is restricted.

EXERCISES

There are many types of exercises for people with chronic back pain, and the choice depends very much on the nature of your particular problem.

Since some exercises may help one type of backache but make another worse, you should be careful when planning your exercise program and discuss any exercises with your physical therapist. The various types of exercises include those already described, aimed at strengthening the back and abdominal muscles (known as isometric exercises), and those that improve movements of the back. It is important to avoid any exercises that make the pain suddenly worse; instead, you should undertake a specific amount of exercise that is gradually increased each day.

AT THE PHYSICAL THERAPIST
A therapy session that involves raising the leg stretches the sciatic nerve.

Exercises for Chronic Back Pain

A simple and safe program of exercises should be undertaken in a graded and gradually increasing fashion. Initially do the following exercises once or twice, then gradually increase up to six times each day as your back allows. For many people, other types of exercises are required, but these should be performed only under the guidance of a physical therapist. Certain exercises can make some types of back pain worse. Much depends on the particular problems in each individual case.

EXERCISE 1

Lie flat on your back on the floor with a pillow under your head. Keep your legs straight and lift each heel in turn, just off the floor. Repeat.

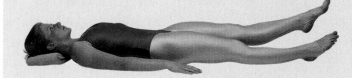

EXERCISE 2

Lie flat on your back on the floor with a pillow under your head. Fold your arms. Lift your head and shoulders just off the floor and then lie flat and relax. Repeat.

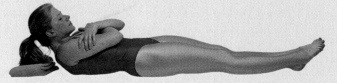

EXERCISE 3

Lie flat on your back on the floor with a pillow under your head. Tense your stomach muscles and flatten the small of your back onto the floor, then relax. Repeat.

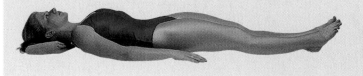

Exercises for Chronic Back Pain (cont'd.)

EXERCISE 4   Lie flat on your back. Reach down the side of one thigh toward your knee. Straighten up and repeat on the other side. Repeat.

Seen from above.

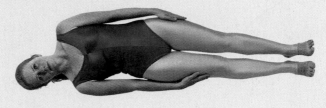

EXERCISE 5   **STEP 1** Lie flat on your back on the floor with a pillow under your head. Bend your knees so that your feet are flat on the ground.

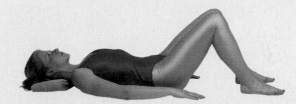

STEP 2 Lift your bottom in the air by tightening your stomach muscles, keeping the back straight. Repeat.

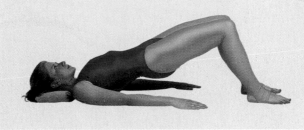

Exercises for Chronic Back Pain (cont'd.)

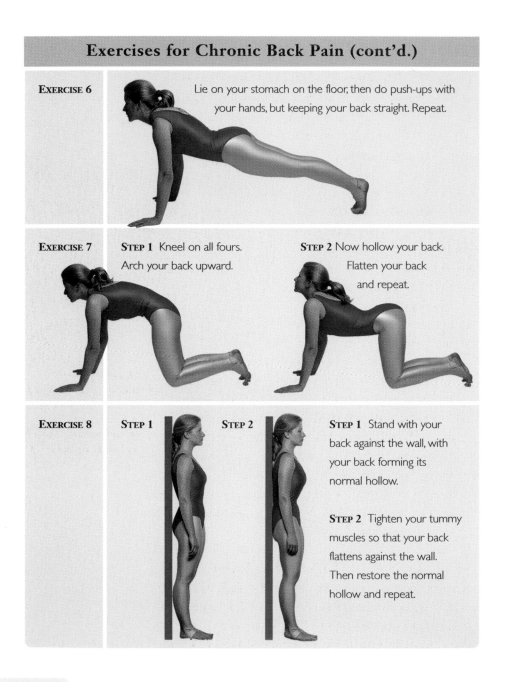

EXERCISE 6

Lie on your stomach on the floor, then do push-ups with your hands, but keeping your back straight. Repeat.

EXERCISE 7

STEP 1 Kneel on all fours. Arch your back upward.

STEP 2 Now hollow your back. Flatten your back and repeat.

EXERCISE 8

STEP 1

STEP 2

STEP 1 Stand with your back against the wall, with your back forming its normal hollow.

STEP 2 Tighten your tummy muscles so that your back flattens against the wall. Then restore the normal hollow and repeat.

SPORTS

You should remain active and return to sports activities as soon as possible after a bout of severe pain. The safest options are walking, swimming, and bicycling. Contact sports such as football are risky because sudden unexpected and forceful movements can undo several weeks of gradual improvement.

MOBILIZATION AND MANIPULATION

There is wide variety between the techniques practiced by physical therapists, osteopaths, chiropractors, physicians, and orthopedic surgeons. Some manipulators apply forces directly to the vertebrae in the spine, whereas others use your shoulders and pelvis as levers.

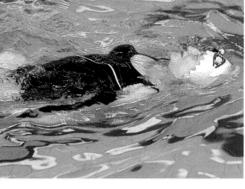

RETURNING TO SPORTS
People who are used to regular exercise should return to sports as soon as possible once their back pain has subsided. Swimming is one of the best and safest forms of exercise for back problems.

There is no agreement among various practitioners on the types of problems for which manipulation is useful, when the different types of manipulation should be used, and the relative usefulness of these treatments.

Manipulation can hasten your recovery from an acute episode of back pain, but it is doubtful that it provides real benefit for chronic back pain. In general, manipulation appears to be safe, although a few people find that it makes their back problems worse.

DRUG TREATMENTS

The primary purpose of drug treatment is to relieve pain. The two main types of drugs used are pure pain relievers, which are known as analgesics, and those that also control inflammation in the area of damage, known as anti-inflammatory drugs. The character of the back problem is often helpful in indicating which type of drug will provide the most effective treatment.

ANALGESICS

Acetaminophen is the most commonly used analgesic. You can take up to six or eight 500-milligram pills a day, and it is safe provided that you do not exceed this dose. You can buy acetaminophen from drugstores without a prescription. There are several stronger analgesics, such as propoxyphene and hydrocodone, which are often combined with acetaminophen, but these are available only by prescription and may be habit-forming.

ANTI-INFLAMMATORY DRUGS

You will find these drugs particularly helpful if you are very stiff in bed and when you wake up in the morning. Their main role is to reduce inflammation, but they are effective analgesics as well. Aspirin was the first anti-inflammatory drug, but it can cause indigestion and abdominal upsets. Larger doses may give you ringing noises in your ears and interfere with your hearing. Ibuprofen and naproxen are available over the counter in pharmacies and seem to produce far fewer problems.

There are alternative anti-inflammatory drugs available by prescription, such as naproxen, diclofenac, piroxicam, ketoprofen, and many others, which are generally taken in pill form. A lot of research has gone into producing newer versions that need to be taken only once or twice a day rather than every few hours.

All anti-inflammatory drugs can cause abdominal upset and you may be prescribed an antiulcer treatment at the same time. Some of the newer anti-inflammatory drugs, such as celecoxib and rofecoxib, have a lower risk of causing stomach problems. If the anti-inflammatory pills upset your digestive system too much, your doctor can prescribe the drug in suppository form. Many insurance and prescription plans strictly limit coverage of the newest medications.

MUSCLE RELAXANTS
If you are one of those people who develop severe spasms of the back muscles, which can be extremely painful, you may find that muscle relaxants are helpful.

ANTICONVULSANT DRUGS
Neuropathic pains are sudden electric shock sensations shooting from the back down the leg, often accompanied by painful tingling and numbness. These seem to result from oversensitivity of the damaged nerves. People with epilepsy have oversensitive brain cells, which fire off in an uncontrolled, random way, causing them to have seizures. The same drugs that are used to control epileptic seizures can also be effective in relieving neuropathic pain.

TRICYCLIC ANTIDEPRESSANTS
Some people who have chronic back problems develop widespread pain; sometimes even their skin becomes so hypersensitive that it is tender to the slightest pressure. Alteration in the pain-processing system in the central nervous system probably underlies this. This type of pain is not helped by conventional analgesics. There may be similar biochemical changes in the central nervous systems of people who are clinically depressed, and the drugs used for treating depression, such as amitriptyline, can be effective for treating this kind of pain.

INJECTIONS

Injections can be very helpful for certain types of back pain. They take a number of different forms depending on the precise nature of the problem.

● **For tender spots** Some people with back problems have one or two very localized tender areas in the back, perhaps in the superficial tissues, in the ligaments connecting the vertebrae, in the sacroiliac joints, or elsewhere. Your doctor can identify the painful areas by feeling your back carefully while you are lying flat in a relaxed position. The tender spots may then be treated with an injection of a small amount of local anesthetic and a steroid, such as cortisone. Steroids also have long-lasting anti-inflammatory action. After the injection, you will usually be pain-free for 2–3 hours due to the anesthetic, then the pain may return for 24 hours or so. However, after that period some people find that the pain diminishes dramatically. This relief varies considerably from one person to another, but for many the pain relief is long-lasting. Cortisone, used intermittently and sparingly in this way, does not cause the degree of adverse effects that may develop when it is taken regularly by mouth.

● **Facet joint injections** The facet joints at the back of the spine can also be treated by means of an injection using a fine needle. It is usually done under X-ray guidance so that the injection can be positioned in precisely the right place in the joint.

● **Epidural injections** An epidural injection is given into the spine around the linings surrounding the spinal cord and nerve roots. Local anesthetic with a small amount of a cortisone-like drug is injected. You may be offered this treatment if you have radiculopathy, or sciatica, that has improved after a severe attack but has not cleared up completely.

— COMPLEMENTARY TREATMENTS —
Some people find that their back pain responds well to complementary treatments such as acupuncture.

ACUPUNCTURE
Back pain can be very difficult to control. Sometimes the symptoms are relieved by blocking the passage of nerve impulses up the spine to the brain.

Acupuncture was first developed in China between 2,000 and 3,000 years ago. It was thought to work by altering the balance between the two opposing life forces known as yin and yang. Acupuncture is at times used in Western medicine today. We now know that it stimulates the release of natural chemicals (known as endorphins and enkephalins) within the brain and spinal cord, which can block the passage of the pain sensations. Sterile needles are inserted through the skin and then rotated to produce stimulation. Some acupuncturists use the traditional Chinese acupuncture sites, but for many this is out of custom rather than belief.

Acupuncture does not work on everybody. Some people respond well, while others derive only short-term benefit and need repeated treatment.

TENS TREATMENT
The problem with acupuncture is that inserting needles through the skin and applying stimulation is a highly skilled technique, and you will have to go to a special practitioner to have it done. TENS (which is the abbreviation for transcutaneous electrical nerve stimulation),

ACUPUNCTURE NEEDLES
Acupuncture, a method of pain relief that involves inserting fine needles into particular points on the body, may be used as a complementary treatment for back pain.

on the other hand, is a treatment that you can do for yourself at home.

To use the TENS technique, you attach electric pads coated with a special electrical conducting jelly to the skin of your back. These are then connected to a battery and stimulator, which can be worn on a belt or in a pocket. When you switch the TENS unit on, multiple tiny pulses of electricity stimulate your skin. You can adjust the strength, frequency, and length of time of each impulse.

USING A TENS MACHINE
The electrical pads of a TENS machine are applied directly to the back. Your doctor or physical therapist will show you how to use this equipment.

The electrical stimulation feels like a tiny prickling sensation in your skin. It acts in a way similar to acupuncture by stimulating nerves, and it releases substances in the brain and spinal cord that block the sensation of back pain.

This technique is useful for anyone with chronic back pain; the stimulator can be switched on whenever the user needs it. As with acupuncture, TENS does not help everyone, but, if you have persistent pain, you should discuss this treatment with your doctor. In some cases, this treatment can be remarkably successful.

BACK BRACE

The lumbar support, or back brace, is a firm body belt extending from the rib cage to the pelvis. It holds strengtheners, behind which may be flat steel strips molded to the shape of your back.

Wearing a lumbar support limits your back movements and increases the pressure within your abdomen and therefore may relieve back pain.

Unfortunately, wearing a back brace for a long time can lead to permanent back stiffness, and in the long run many back braces do as much harm as good.

We now believe that, for most people, the aim should be to restore movements to the back as soon as possible, which is the reason that braces are now used only rarely.

SURGICAL TREATMENTS

Only about one operation is needed for every 2,000 attacks of back pain. Surgery should be considered only if your symptoms have not responded to treatment, if you have severe and persistent pain, and if your problem is of the type likely to improve after an operation. This means that surgery is unlikely to be considered as soon as an attack of back pain develops. Other types of treatment will be tried first, and most people recover without the need for an operation. If you reach the point where an operation is being considered, your surgeon will arrange for detailed tests to be performed. Only certain types of back problems are likely to respond well to surgery. In particular, there are very good results for those who have severe pain in the leg due to nerve compression. On the other hand, the success rate is not nearly as good for those whose main problem is pain in the back itself.

WHICH OPERATION?

There are several different types of back operations. The most common is to remove a herniated disk, most commonly the disk between the fourth and fifth lumbar vertebrae or between the fifth lumbar vertebra and the sacrum. In some cases, the main problem is caused by pressure on the nerve roots from the bone of the vertebral column. The surgeon will try to relieve the pressure by taking away bone to create more space. Sometimes there is excessive movement between the bones of the vertebral column, in which case the surgeon may decide to fuse the vertebrae together. This is known as a spinal fusion.

CONVALESCENCE

After surgery, you will probably start to get up and walk within a few days. You might have to wear a lumbar support for a few weeks, but you may get back to light work within a month or two. It will be several months, however, before you can consider doing any heavy manual work. You should always ask your surgeon before undertaking any activities that might cause excessive stress on your spine.

INTENSIVE REHABILITATION

A small proportion of people with chronic back pain develop very severe symptoms and unfortunately become extremely disabled.

There are a number of reasons for this, including not only the mechanical forms of damage around the spine but also scarring, which may develop around the nerve roots. There may be other changes that can occur within the central nervous system itself, and the whole problem is often exacerbated by depression and anxiety.

Unfortunately, this type of back pain can be very difficult to treat. People in this situation will often need a careful and sympathetic professional assessment of the problem. This will include not only an analysis of the physical problem but also of the patient's reactions to it. The next stage is designing an intensive rehabilitation program tailored to the requirements of the particular individual. This program is intended to restore physical function and help the person to cope with the problem and lead a more normal life.

This type of treatment can be very effective for the most severely disabled back sufferers. It is available in inpatient rehabilitation facilities and some chronic pain centers.

KEY POINTS

- Your medical history and clinical examination are the most important parts of assessment. Imaging tests are a useful supplement in appropriate cases.
- The back sufferer should understand how the back works, what goes wrong, and why various types of treatment are used.
- Exercise is good for the back, but sudden forceful movements should be avoided.
- The choice of medication is related to the clinical problem. Most pain can be controlled by a simple painkiller such as acetaminophen, or anti-inflammatory drugs such as ibuprofen.
- Intensive rehabilitation programs are effective for people with severe chronic back problems.

Useful addresses

There are several national societies that are concerned with the welfare of people with back pain and with raising funds for research into better methods of diagnosis and treatment. Several of these organizations produce helpful booklets that provide useful factual information.

American Association of Retired Persons (AARP)
Online: www.aarp.org
601 E Street NW
Washington, DC 20049
Tel: (800) 424-3410
Tel: (877) 434-7598 (TTY)
E-mail: member@aarp.org

Foundation for Osteoporosis Research and Education
Online: www.fore.org
300 27th Street, Suite 103
Oakland, CA 94612
Tel: (888) 266-3015
Tel: (510) 832-2663

National Institute of Arthritis and Musculoskeletal and Skin Diseases
Online: www.nih.gov/niams
National Institute of Health
1 AMS Circle
Bethesda, MD 20892
Tel: (301) 496-8188
Tel: (301) 565-2966 (TTY)
E-mail: niamsic@mail.nih/gov

National Osteoporosis Foundation
Online: www.nof.org
1150 17th Street NW
Washington, DC 20036-4603
Tel: (800) 223-9994
Tel: (202) 223-2226
E-mail: nofmail@nof.org

Older Women's League (OWL)
Online: www.owl-national.com
666 11th Street NW, Suite 700
Washington, DC 20001
Tel: (202) 783-6686

Osteoporosis and Related Bone Diseases National Resource Center (ORBD-NRC)
Online: www.osteo.org
1150 17th Street NW
Washington, DC 20036-4603
Tel: (800) 624-BONE
Tel: (202) 223-0344
Tel: (202) 466-4315 (TTY)
E-mail: orbdnrc@nof.org

University of California's Ostcoporosis and Arthritis Research Group (UCSF-OARG)
350 Parnassus Avenue
Box 1349
San Francisco, CA 94143-1349

Notes

Notes

Notes

Index

Acknowledgments

PUBLISHER'S ACKNOWLEDGMENTS
Dorling Kindersley Publishing, Inc. would like to thank the following for their help and participation in this project:

Managing Editor Stephanie Jackson; **Managing Art Editor** Nigel Duffield; **Editorial Assistance** Judit Z. Bodnar, Mary Lindsay, Jennifer Quasha, Ashley Ren, Design Revolution; **Design Assistance** Sarah Hall, Design Revolution, Chris Walker; **Production** Michelle Thomas, Elizabeth Cherry.

Consultancy Dr. Tony Smith, Dr. Sue Davidson; **Indexing** Indexing Specialists, Hove; **Administration** Christopher Gordon.

Organizations St. John's Ambulance, St. Andrew's Ambulance Organization, British Red Cross.

Illustrations (p.12, p.13, p.14, p.20, p.22, p.23) © Philip Wilson.

Picture Research Angela Anderson, Andy Sansom; **Picture Librarian** Charlotte Oster.

PICTURE CREDITS
The publisher would like to thank the following for their kind permission to reproduce their photographs. Every effort has been made to trace the copyright holders. Dorling Kindersley apologizes for any unintentional omissions and would be pleased, in any such cases, to add an acknowledgment in future editions.

APM Studios p.60, p.61, p.62; **Sally & Richard Greenhill Photo Library** p.9, p.63; **Institute of Orthopaedics** p.57; **Science Photo Library** p.19 (Keene/BSIP), p.30 (Sheila Terry), p.47 (BSIP, Ducloux), p.52 (Professor P. Motta), p.57 (Jerome Yeats), p.58 (Tirot/BSIP).